Contents

Introduction	1
Glossary	3
History	5
The Quest for Plate Spinning (Figuring it out for Myself)	7
A Note on the Method…	9
Different Techniques for Plate Spinning	11
Things to Look for in a "Plate"	15
Shop Talk	21
Building a Plate Spinning Rack	23
Technique	33
And so, We Begin…	35
Other Techniques	39
Troubleshooting	43
Big Finish	47
Notes on Performance	49
Tool Kit for Plate Spinning	53
Risk Assessment - Plate Spinning	55
Conclusion	57
Special Thanks	59
About the Author	61
Other Books by Modern Vaudeville Press	63

Pottery in Motion:

A practical guide to the impractical art of plate spinning

Sam Veale

Modern Vaudeville Press
PHILADELPHIA, PA

Copyright © 2020 by Sam Veale.

Illustrations by Sorrel Sparks.

Edited by Thom Wall.

All rights reserved. No part of this publication may be reproduced, distributed or transmitted in any form or by any means, including photocopying, recording, or other electronic or mechanical methods, without the prior written permission of the publisher, except in the case of brief quotations embodied in critical reviews and certain other noncommercial uses permitted by copyright law. For permission requests, write to the publisher, addressed "Attention: Permissions Coordinator," at the address below.

Modern Vaudeville Press
Philadelphia, PA
www.ModernVaudevillePress.com

Ordering Information:
Quantity sales. Special discounts are available on quantity purchases by corporations, associations, and others. For details, contact the "Special Sales Department" at the address above.

Plate Spinning / Sam Veale. —1st ed.
ISBN   978-1-7339712-3-2

To my lovely wife Andrianna. I'm sorry I broke one of your blue and white bowls by trying to spin it on a stick. I'm also sorry that I didn't tell you about it and you had to read this book to find out.

Introduction

I LEARNT TO JUGGLE 25 years ago and, shortly after that, I learnt how to spin a toy spinning plate. These specially shaped, soft plastic plates are a favourite at circus skills workshops and learning to spin one on a hand held stick is a minor rite-of-passage for many jugglers. For most however, it ends there.

Some jugglers will go on to use a metal spinning plate as part of a combination trick (a juggling trick where different skills are performed with different parts of the body e.g juggling balls whilst balancing a spinning plate) but these plates, like their plastic counterparts, have a deep dimple in the middle and are not the kind of thing you would find in your kitchen. Very few jugglers learn how to spin real plates and there are several reasons for this.

Firstly, it involves a lot of large, awkward and heavy props. Carrying props around can already be the bane of a juggler's life, so the idea of adding furniture and crockery to an already full kit bag is more than most can bear.

Secondly, these props are not commercially available and have to be specially built by someone who knows how to do so.

And thirdly, there probably isn't anybody around to teach you. I learnt how to juggle mainly from other jugglers. If there was a skill I wanted to learn, I asked somebody who already had that skill. If there was a prop I wanted to try, I could usually borrow it. This wasn't a option with plate spinning. Plate spinners are a rarity and most are professional performers. Asking any professional to reveal the secret of how they do their job can be very awkward, so I had to figure it out for myself.

Glossary

Plate rack - A table or stand of some sort with upward pointing sticks fixed to it for spinning plates on.

Tabletop- The flat surface on top of the plate rack that the sticks are mounted in.

Juggling - Performing art based on the overtly skilful manipulation of inanimate objects. In my opinion, this includes plate spinning.

Launch - The initial move that sets a plate spinning.

Foot / Foot ridge - The raised circular ridge on the base of a plate or bowl that enables it to be spun by holding the tip of the stick in place.

Rescue - Re-accelerate a plate that has slowed and begun to wobble thus preventing it from falling.

Plate - Bowl.

Bowl - Plate.

Pole - A stick that you spin a plate on.

Stick - A pole that you spin a plate on.

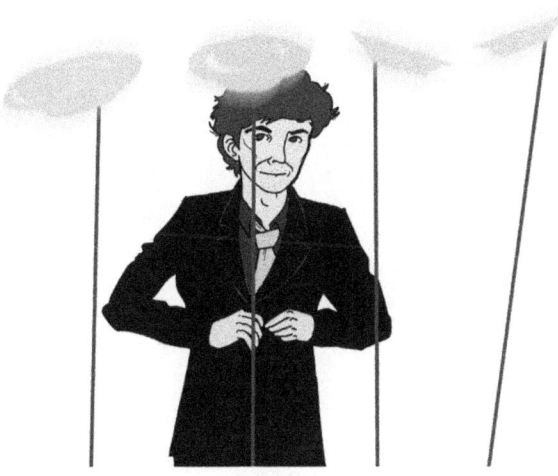

4 | Pottery in Motion:

HISTORY

PLATE SPINNING ORIGINATED in China during the Han Dynasty between 206BC and 220AD.

The Han Dynasty was a period of economic and scientific prosperity. Amongst innovations in such fields as paper-making, they also found time to invent something infinitely less useful - plate spinning.

In Europe, there is no record of plate spinning until about 1000 years later. Oddly enough, you can say the same of paper-making, but I reckon that's just a coincidence. Thinking about it though, I guess they needed to invent paper before they could have a historical record of anything, let alone plate spinning but I doubt they invented paper simply as a means to describe wobbly plates on sticks.

During the Music Hall and Vaudeville era (late 19th to early 20th century), plate spinning became a popular addition to many juggling acts. Many performers were "Salon" jugglers whose act would take place in a domestic setting, or "Gentleman" jugglers who used everyday objects. Plate spinning lent itself to these styles very easily.

Paper was also widely used at this time but that's hardly relevant. I don't know why you keep bringing it up.

By the late 20th century, juggling had ceased to be a skill exclusive to professional performers and was becoming popular amongst hobbyists. Within this community, plate spinning was largely confined to the use of the specially shaped plates mentioned in the introduction. Spinning real plates however, remained largely undiscovered by the new generation of jugglers.

At some point, the term "plate spinning" or "spinning plates" entered the language as a metaphor for things like time management in the office, multi tasking at home or just being very busy. If you Google the phrase "I'm spinning plates" you will be several pages into the search results before you come across anything about plate spinning in the literal sense.

So who invented plate spinning? My favourite theory is that someone was struggling to describe how busy their life was and invented plate spinning just so that they would have something to compare it to. This almost certainly isn't true, but I do like the idea.

The Quest for Plate Spinning (Figuring it out for Myself)

AS I WILL DISCUSS in a later section, there are several different techniques for spinning 'real' plates. Most of these methods involve adapting the plates in some small way to allow the stick or pole to gain purchase on the base of the plate. This is fine, but I was determined to do it with unadapted plates.

Armed with the dangerous combination of curiosity and internet access, I set to work studying photographs and video footage of plate spinners from the past and trying my best to 'back-engineer' the props into something I could build at home. Over the next 18 months I ordered dozens of sticks made of metal, wood, plastic and carbon fibre in a variety of lengths and widths. I massacred pieces of flat-pack furniture and picked the brains of any carpenter, prop builder or metal worker unlucky enough to be on my radar.

It was a difficult process because I had to learn the technique as I worked out how to build the props. If I already had the props, then learning the technique would have been a lot simpler. If I already had the technique, then I would have a much better idea of how to build the rack and of what plates I needed. As it was, I had to piece everything together very slowly. Writing this book is an attempt to give the reader a head start on both learning plate spinning and building the necessary kit.

Pottery in Motion:

A Note on the Method…

THE TECHNIQUES FOR PLATE spinning discussed in this book are based purely on my own research and are by no means definitive. If you choose to pursue this celebrated and ancient art form, you might adapt and build on my experience to create something of your own. Let me know how you get on.

Pottery in Motion:

Different Techniques for Plate Spinning

WHEN I FIRST SET OUT to learn plate spinning, my primary objective was to do it with unadapted, off-the-shelf plates. There are other methods that involve customising the plates in various ways. This book is concerned mainly with unadapted/un-customised plate spinning but it is useful to start with a brief discussion of some of the other methods.

Methods for spinning adapted plates

Tape and spike - A piece of sticky tape (gaffer tape, duct tape or similar) is stuck to the middle of the plate underside. The plate spinning pole (or stick) ends in a sharp spike which pokes into the tape slightly off centre enabling the plate to be driven in circles by rotating the top of the pole.

Washer - A metal washer or ring is glued to the plate underside in the exact centre. The plate is accelerated by tapping the edge (basketball style). The washer can also be placed off centre and the plate accelerated in the same way as the tape and spike method, by rotating the pole.

Drilled plate - Similar to the central washer method but a shallow hole is drilled into the plate instead of the washer. Can also be drilled off centre (see 'washer,' above).

Advantages of adapted plate techniques

- A wide range of plates can be adapted and used. This means that you can travel with just the plate rack and buy plates at your destination. Especially useful when working abroad.
- When spinning, the plates are relatively stable and have a good spin time so more plates can be spun. An adapted plate method was used to set the world record at a staggering 108 plates (David Spathaky, Bangkok, Thailand, 1996).

Disadvantages

- The plates don't wobble as much as with other techniques. The classic appeal of plate spinning is the jeopardy of the plate on the verge of falling, so this method can be a bit less visual.
- It is often performed with the plates at waist level or not much higher. Not really a disadvantage so much as an aesthetic choice, but a higher plate is more visual and looks more dangerous.
- Getting the pole into the right spot on the plate can be fiddly. If the performer looks like they are 'threading the needle' when they place each new plate, it can look rigged and unconvincing.
- Adapting the plates is cheating??? (see below)

Cheating???

Some performers adapt their plates to such an extent that the whole trick is essentially self working. Hand held sticks attached to bearings glued to the base of a metal plate is one example of this. But is it cheating to adapt the plates?

Plate spinning is not a sport. There are no rules, so I guess there is no such thing as cheating, but an audience would be unlikely to see it that way if they spot you using a gimmick. In reality, they probably won't notice and if the show is entertaining they won't care, but I was determined to be a purist about plate spinning. How you feel about your own material is just as important as how a spectator might feel about it and this is just the way that I wanted to do it. I use adapted, everyday objects for some other juggling and balancing tricks, but for some reason, I wanted to plate spin with plain and simple plates. I've also found that, after learning the "pure" method, adapted methods are relatively easy to pick up.

Unadapted plate method

A plate with a well defined, circular ridge on the base is spun on a pole that comes to a point. The point is held inside the ridge and the plate is accelerated by rapidly rotating the base of the pole.

Advantages

- Wobble! The plates and especially the poles have more movement. This makes them look less stable which is more dramatic and visual.
- Taller. Plate racks for this method tend to be taller with the plates above eye level. This is arguably more visual.
- Not "cheating." Again, highly debatable. It's up to you.

Disadvantages

- Only specific plates can be used. Suitable plates can be difficult to find and replace. This can lead to a lot of shopping around.

14 | Pottery in Motion:

THINGS TO LOOK FOR IN A "PLATE"

OK, I ADMIT IT. I've been lying to you. I don't spin plates, I spin bowls.

I know!

Shocking!

This far into the book and I drop a bombshell like that.

The term "Bowl Spinner" doesn't have the same ring about it or the same cultural significance as "Plate Spinner" but it is more accurate. The type of "plates" I recommend are variously called "soup bowls," "pasta bowls" or "deep dish plates" (See! they are called plates sometimes).

My early experiments into plate spinning did involve using regular dinner plates but I moved onto deep dish plates for a couple of very good reasons. They are taller than a regular plate which makes them wobble more dramatically, and they have a smaller "foot" (see below).

Foot Fetish

Whenever I'm in a restaurant or cafe, I reach under the plate of food I've ordered and feel the ridge on the base of the plate. This ridge is called the "foot" and it enables the plate to be glazed in a kiln without any of the glaze touching the kiln wall and ruining the finish (it's amazing what you learn in this line of work!). The shape of this ridge, determines whether the plate can be spun.

When I examine the inside of this ridge, I'm asking myself three questions:
- How deep is it?
- How steep is it? And...
- Will the waiter notice if I steal it? (n.b It's probably best to take a photo of the brand name on the base and look it up online later. You get banned from fewer restaurants that way)

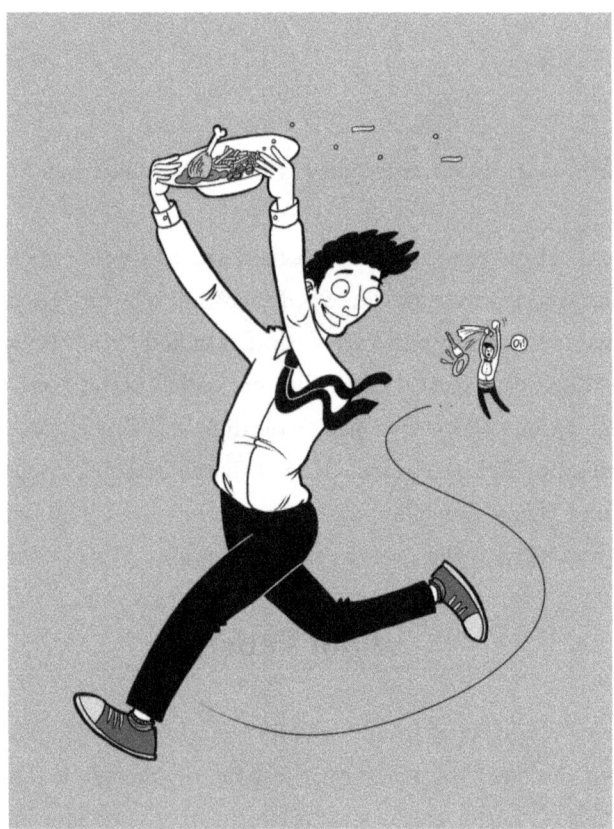

It is this ridge that will hold the tip of the pole when the plate is spinning. Without a well defined ridge, the plate cannot be spun.

Things to Look for in a "Plate" | 17

A - Shallow ridge - Some plates barely have a ridge at all. This is a cross section of an unsuitable plate. This plate would not work at all except possibly at a very slow speed

B - Deeper ridge - This one would work but the angle is a bit shallow so it might fall when accelerated to a higher speed.

C - Steep ridge - This ridge is deeper than the one above and the angle is steeper. In fact, the angle is more important than the depth and will enable the point to hold the plate even at high speed.

D - Steep, deep ridge - This ridge is as steep as the one above but is deeper. The depth makes no difference to how fast it can be spun but it will be more stable when launched or when rescued from a very slow wobble.

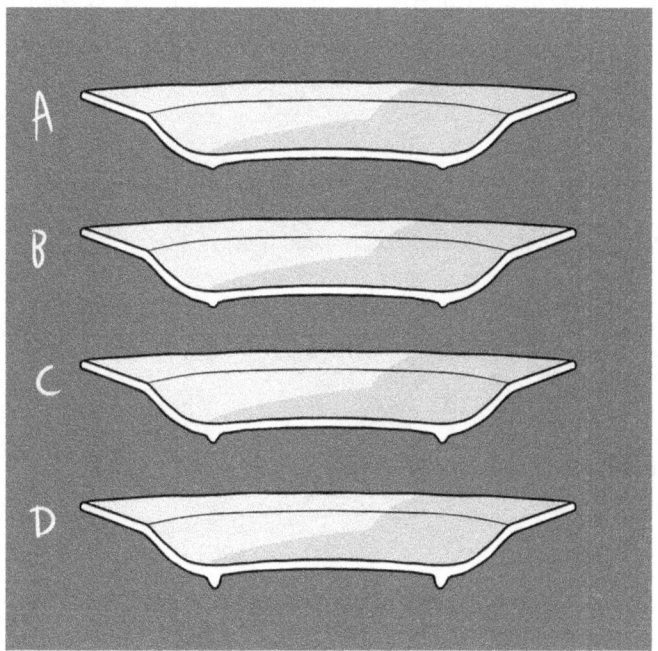

Foot Diameter

Another important factor is the diameter of the foot. As I mentioned earlier, the first plates I used were large dinner plates. They had a nice steep ridge which held the point of the stick really well, but the foot was 15cm (6 inches) across. They were usable but the large diameter meant that it took a long time to get them back up to speed once they had started to slow down. My current plates (Bowls? Whatever!) have a foot that is 8.5cm (3 & 1/4 inches) in diameter and can be rescued (re-accelerated) a lot more quickly.

Imagine swinging a 10 foot rope in a circle over your head. You would have to start it off with a very big, slow movement and accelerate from there. Now imagine doing the same thing with 5 foot rope. You get up to full speed a lot more quickly. Spinning a plate is the same basic principle. You don't want the foot diameter to be too small though as the pole wobble will be reduced and might be less visual.

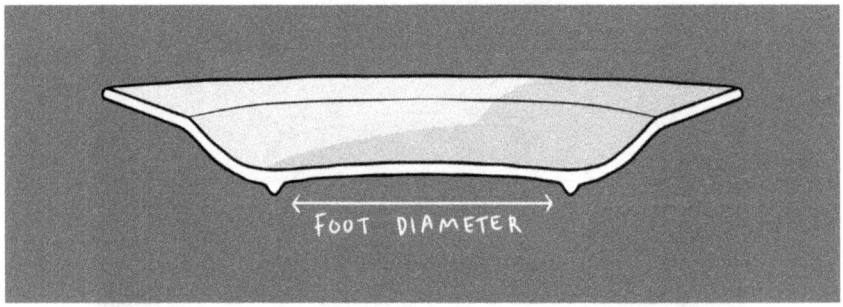

Alternatively, use plastic plates

By this, I don't mean toy spinning plates. If you shop around, you might find some melamine (or similar) plates that are similar to their ceramic counterparts and have a good foot as described above. This is great to get you started but china plates will be probably be heavier and hence, spin for longer, so switch up to them as soon as you feel able. Even when you are rehearsing.

20 | Pottery in Motion:

Shop Talk

I CAN'T TELL YOU where to buy plates, but hopefully, the above guidelines will help you find what you're looking for with some shopping around.

The first deep dish plates I used were part of the budget crockery range from a chain of shops in the UK. This was perfect as they were cheap and widely available so I bought about 30. I could have bought more, but I was new to plate spinning and thought I might find something better. Besides, these plates were easy to find and I could always get spares unless the whole chain went bust and closed down… which is exactly what happened.

I suspended my practice schedule for fear of breaking my few remaining plates and went on a shopping spree. I bought one of every suitable looking plate I could find in my local area. At the end of the day, I had about a dozen candidates that I auditioned at home. The plate audition involved spinning each one as fast as I could and timing how long it took to fall. In actual fact, I didn't let them fall as I had kept the receipts and wanted to get my money back, but I let them spin until I could tell they were about to go.

There was a clear winner, so I went back to the shop (another national chain) and discovered that the favourite was from a discontinued line and they only had a couple more in stock. There were several other branches of this shop in my area, so I went to all of them and bought the few remaining plates but I still only had about 15 (I spin 8 in the show, but spares are reassuring).

Luckily, I had a show coming up about 150 miles from my house. I mapped every branch of this shop along the way and visited all of them in search of the last remaining plates. By the end of what has to be the

22 | Pottery in Motion:

most pathetic UK tour of all time, I had more than enough plates to feel comfortable using them in the show.

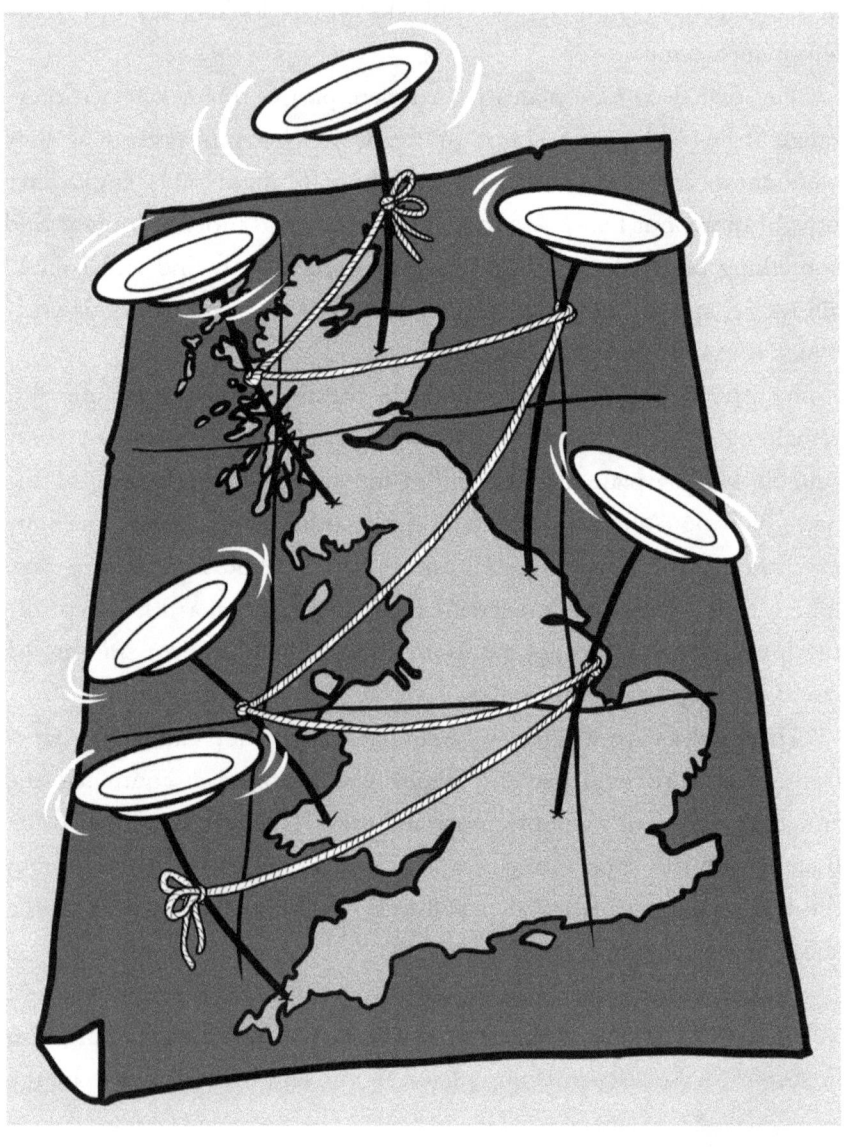

BUILDING A PLATE SPINNING RACK

THIS BOOK DOES NOT contain precise plans on how to build your own plate rack. This would not be practical as some of the parts were custom made for me. Other parts were off the shelf, but from specific suppliers who cannot be relied on to keep exactly the same stock.

Instead of exact plans, what follows is a description of my own racks and the principles I followed that are important to their function.

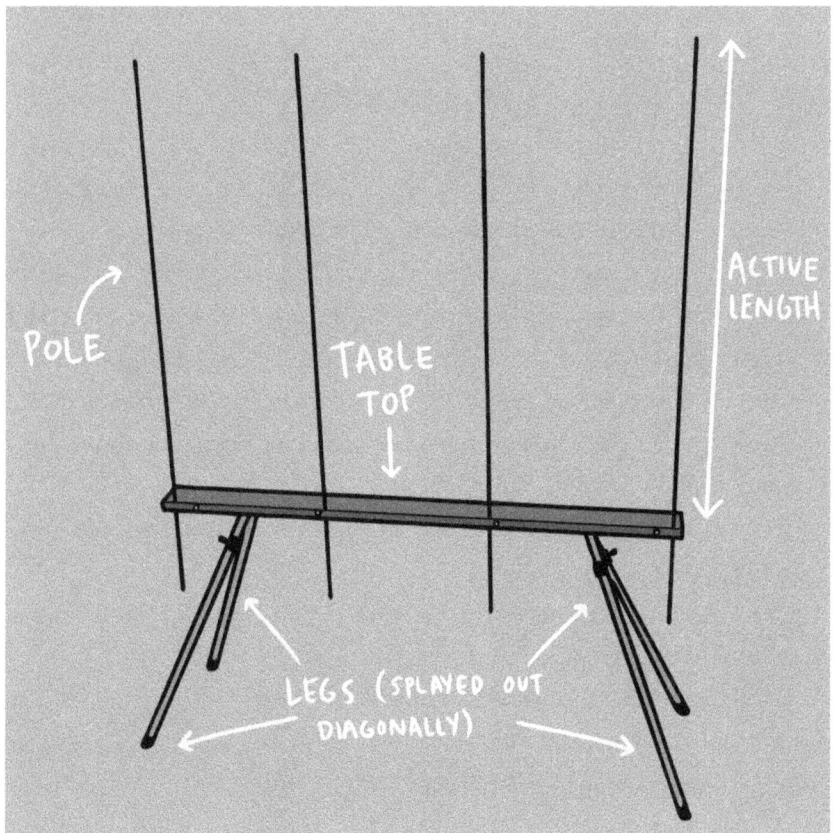

Basic Principles

A plate rack must be…

- Solid - If it wobbles when the plates are spinning, they will slow down more quickly (the wobble is kinetic energy leaking out of the system rather than staying in the plates). Also, rescuing a plate that is on a wobbly rack is more difficult.
- Portable - It doesn't need to be feather light but it does need to be carried, and travelled with. It should be collapsible to some extent as well (Removable legs etc).
- Wide Enough to store plates - Remember, during your show, you will need somewhere to put the plates before and after you spin them. Your rack needs to operate as a table unless you want to keep the plates elsewhere.

Practice Rig

Before I built a full rack, I built a simple, makeshift, one-pole practice rig to learn the technique and experiment with different plates/poles etc.

I drilled a hole in a piece of wood and clamped it, firmly to a garden table. I pushed a stick into the hole and used it as a one plate rack. This is a crude but effective way that you can try different lengths and types of pole and you can time the plate to see how long it takes to slow down. Practising with a scaled down rig like this will tell you a lot about using a larger rig.

Remember, the stick should fit very tightly so that it does not move around inside the hole at all.

More recently, I've been using a work bench with adjustable jaws at the top to clamp the pole into place.

It's a good idea to master spinning one plate like this before you build a full rig. This way, you know that you have the right plate/stick combination to apply to the full rack.

Building a Plate Spinning Rack | 25

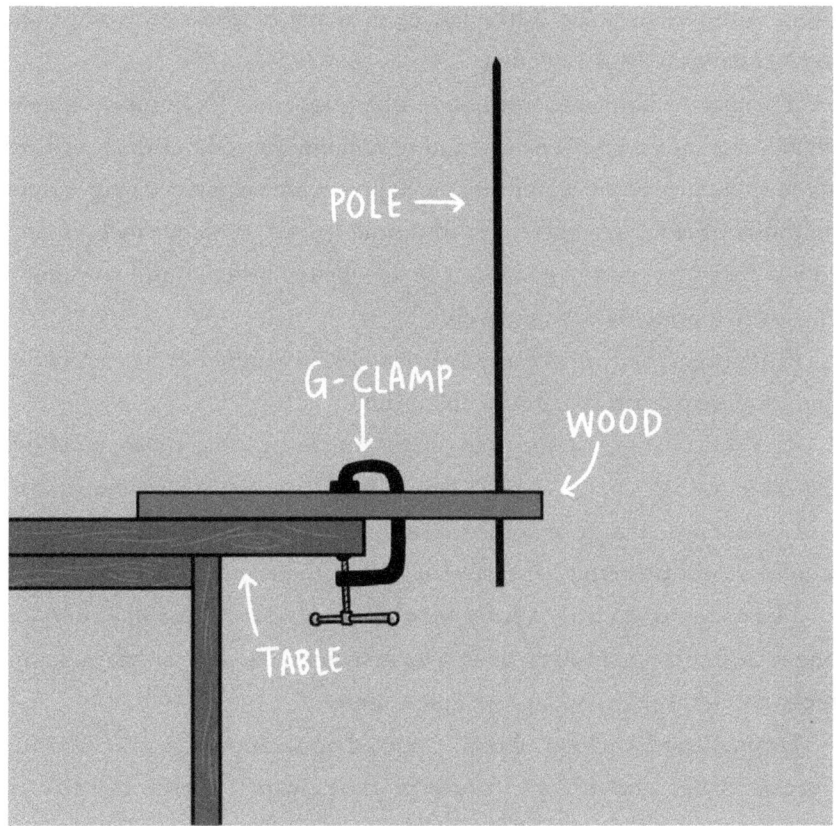

After this, my first prototype plate spinning rack involved two trestles from a furniture shop and a lot of g-clamps. It worked, but moving it even a short distance across the floor was difficult and clumsy. I knew I needed something better. This is how I did it. It is not the only way. Not by any means, but it does work and I hope you will find it a useful starting point.

Poles (sticks)

These are the poles that your plates will actually spin on. I have a garage full of wooden dowels, metal poles, plastic sticks, carbon fibre tubes and garden poles. Although I got many of these to work, none performed exactly as I needed.

The best results came from using fibreglass rods. Eight millimetres in diameter to be precise. The six- and ten millimetre rods work as well but eight millimetre rod was, for me, the happy medium. After trying various methods of adapting the tip of the pole (metal, rubber, vinyl ends), I found that very simply putting it in a pencil sharpener and working it almost to a point works very well.

Warning: This will destroy the pencil sharpener. Buy several cheap ones and be prepared to chuck them out.

The active length of the pole (that is, the length that sticks out above the table top of the rack) is 121cm. The poles I use are 150cm in total so I can adjust this to be longer or shorter if need be. Different active lengths might be better for different plates. Experiment!

I have two racks with 4 poles on each. I could have put all 8 poles on one rack but it would have been a lot less portable unless the 'tabletop' section could fold in half or be taken apart.

Important: Don't get fibreglass mixed up with carbon fibre. Carbon fibre is stiffer and usually comes in tubes which therefore can't be sharpened to a point. Carbon fibre can be made to work if you can fashion a tip or use narrow ones. I did experiment with 5.3mm tubes for a while (in fact, these were the first poles I managed to spin a real plate on). They worked but I managed to break one or two of them at the joint with the rack. This has never happened with fibre glass.

I have heard of other plate spinners using tempered aluminium or flexible wooden dowels.

Experiment!

Adapting the Tips

Mostly, I have been working with poles that are simply sharpened as described above. In an early experiment, I used a soft vinyl end cap on the tip of the stick. This was great for grip and acceleration but the plate slowed down very quickly making it unusable.

The following adaptation however, can provide extra grip on the base of the plate and extend spin time.

Step 1 - Carefully drill a narrow hole into the end of the stick exactly in the centre.

Step 2 - Cut the head off a nail and insert it all the way into the hole with the point facing upwards. Be careful not to split the stick. Superglue it in if it doesn't fit tightly.

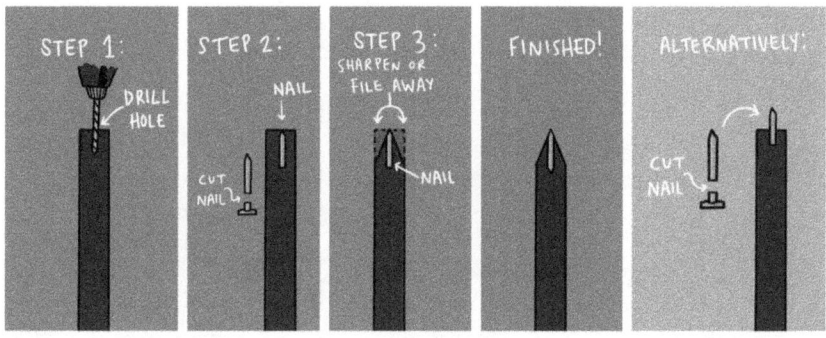

Step 3 - Sharpen the end of the stick with a pencil sharpener until the sharpener gets to the metal of the nail.

Alternatively, you can just cut the head off a nail and insert it point upwards into the hole so that it sticks out about 1cm above the top of the stick.

In Colour (Color)

Ideally, the poles should be a different colour to the plates. A contrasting colour makes them look more like separate pieces and not like they are stuck on. You might also consider some reflective sticky tape on the poles to catch the stage light and flash when wobbling.

Tabletop

This is the bit that the poles will stick into. The poles need to be held in place very firmly so that there is no play at the base of the pole (i.e., they don't move around in the hole they are in). There are any number of ways you could achieve this. I hit upon a relatively simple solution but it isn't the only one.

My tabletop is made of two pieces of pine, both 150cm long and 2.6cm (1 inch) high.

The larger piece (that the legs are attached to) is 8cm wide and the smaller piece is 1.5cm wide.

The two pieces are tightly bolted together lengthways with 100mm bolts and the holes (for the sticks) are drilled exactly on the join between

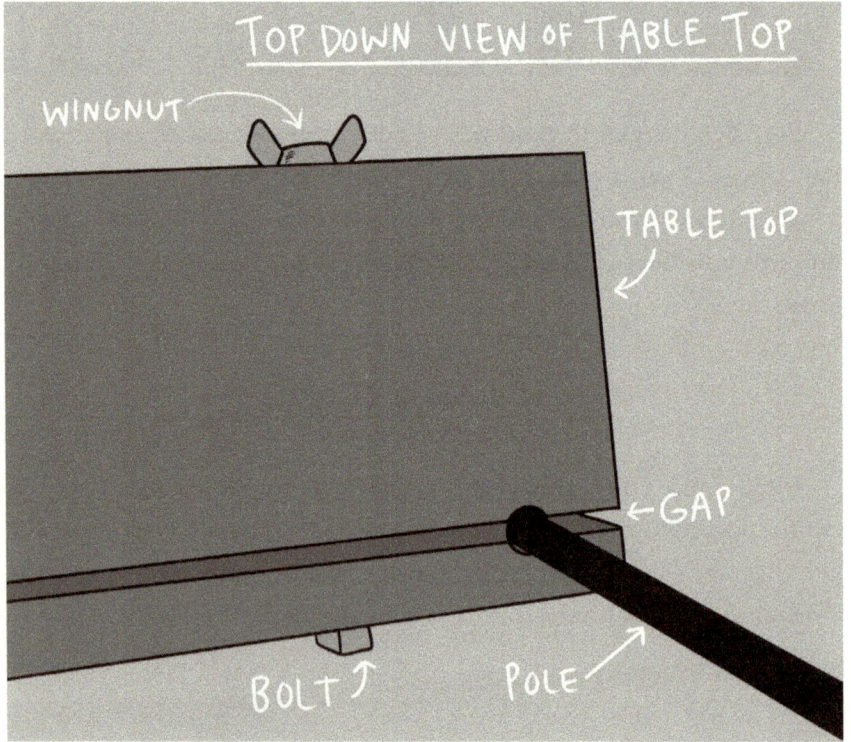

the two pieces of wood. When you unbolt the wood the hole is looser and the poles can be easily fitted and tightened into place.

The holes are evenly spaced along the join. In my case they are at 48cm intervals (3cm, 51cm, 99cm and 147cm). If the poles are too close together they might sway and cause the plates to crash into one another.

Use a pillar drill (drill press) not a hand drill to make the holes for the sticks. Alternatively, you could also use a drill guide. This will ensure that they are exactly vertical. If a pole is slightly off vertical, it will still work but may be more unstable and slow more quickly.

Important: The holes should be drilled slightly smaller than the diameter of the poles. You can buy drill bits in decimal point sizes. I used a 7.8mm drill bit to make holes for the 8mm poles. This ensured a tight fit.

The poles are tightened into place with wing-nuts but I use a wrench to get them extra tight.

Record Breaker

A few months ago, I arrived at a venue later than planned after getting stuck in traffic. Whilst I was in plenty of time for the start of the show, my set-up procedure had to be hurried. This is exactly the kind of situation where it's easy to make mistakes, and the mistake I made was forgetting to tighten the bolts that hold the poles in place. I had remembered to tighten them by hand but forgotten to use the wrench to get them extra tight. My plate spinning routine was about 40 minutes into the 45 minute show so it was some time before I realised my mistake. Plates that usually span quite happily for over a minute were slowing down after less than 30 seconds. By the end of the show I had broken 5 of them. A new record! (n.b. The previous record was 4. See below.)

I always keep 4 plates hidden on stage as spares but the 5 breakages had left me with only 7 plates and 8 poles. When I finally had them all spinning, I triumphantly announced to the audience:

"All unbroken plates spinning at the same time!!!"

The great thing about plate spinning is that it's just as entertaining when it goes badly wrong.

Arguably more so.

Legs

The legs should be splayed diagonally outwards from each corner of the rack. This adds to the stability and helps allow longer spin times. On my setup, the legs are splayed out about 23 degrees lengthways and about 16 degrees out to the sides (from vertical).

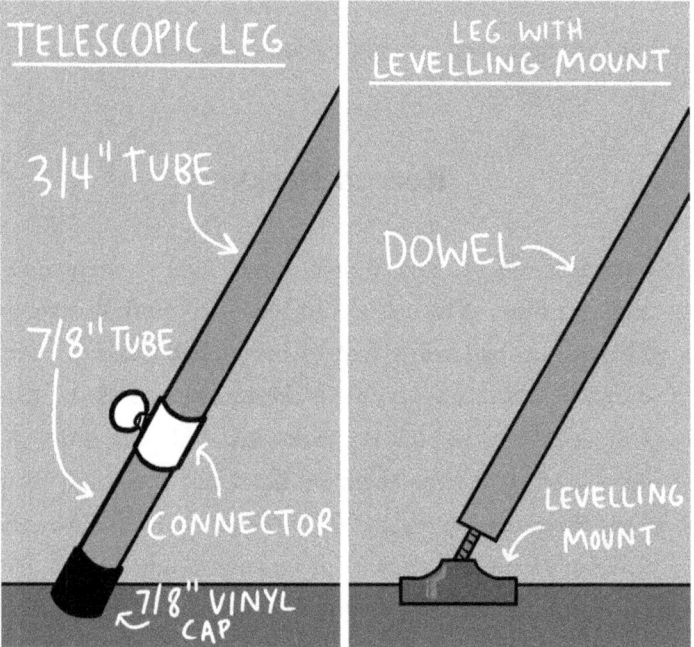

Bear in mind that splayed out legs can be a trip hazard. Make sure they are clearly visible or well out of the way when not in use.

I made the legs from telescopic steel tubing using 3/4", 7/8" and 1" diameter tube (The tubes fit inside one another snugly). Short sections of the 1" tubes were welded to the baseplates (leg holders). Most of the leg length was the 7/8" tube and the 3/4" length was added to the end to make it adjustable for uneven surfaces (Search for telescopic tubing kit online).

Another option is to use adjustable table feet (Levelling mounts). These can screw into the end of a dowel and be tightened or loosened to stop wobbling on uneven floors.

This last point is very important. If the legs are not adjustable then the plate rack will wobble on an uneven surface and the plates will slow down more quickly (see "Basic Principles" above).

Spirit Level (aka a level)

Along with a dustpan and brush, you'll also want to carry a spirit level in your kit bag. The table top of your rig doesn't have to be perfectly horizontal but it can be useful to have a visual guide to get it as close as possible especially if you are working on a raked stage or uneven ground.

Leg Baseplates

These I had specially made by a welder using short lengths of 1" tubing to a metal baseplate about 8cm square. This is the only part I had to have custom made. A similar solution made in wood or another material would work just as well, as long as it is not too flexible and the legs are splayed as described above.

Weights

For extra stability you can hang weights from the bottom of the rack. Rather than carrying heavy weights around with you, use water tanks (large water bottles) and hang them from a hook under the middle of the rack.

Full Length Stick

I experimented briefly with 2 metre (6 & 1/2 ft) poles that extended from a low rack on the floor. This worked but I had to stoop down to hold the pole in the best position for accelerating the plate which looked and felt very awkward.

Technique

Safety First

IT IS WORTH CONSIDERING safety before you start working on your technique. Not just your own safety, but that of anyone else sharing your practice space. Sorry if this just sounds like common sense but I'd rather mention it than not.

A Few Points to Remember

Broken plates can have VERY sharp edges (even plastic, melamine plates). They can also break into tiny pieces so...

- Don't practise barefoot or just in socks (this is also because plates are heavy and might land on your feet!)
- Tidy up very thoroughly if you have a breakage - Vacuum if you can.
- Put broken pieces into a separate bag before putting them in the bin.

Breakages can be avoided by...

- Practising on a lawn.
- Covering the floor with some kind of padding (exercise mat etc.)
- Covering the rack with some kind of padding (the plate might hit the rack on the way down.)

Bear in mind that none of this will help if one plate falls and another lands on top of it so you might want to… Use plastic plates (see plate buying guide above,) although even these can break. Just be careful!

Where to Practise

This has been a problem for me since I started plate spinning. A plate spinning rack is an awkward thing to take to your local juggling club and it takes up so much space that you can no longer glare judgementally at club passers, unicyclists and poi spinners for hogging the room. It might be an option but it depends on available space and the goodwill of your fellow jugglers (who will probably all want to have a go!). Breaking plates could make you unpopular too.

Not everyone is lucky enough to have a garden. Using the the garden can make rehearsing a seasonal affair and even a light breeze can slow plates down prematurely. Indoors might be possible depending on the height of your rack and the patience of your family/housemates/downstairs neighbours etc…

What I'm trying to say is think about where and how you will rehearse before you go to the trouble of building a plate rack. It is not the most convenient form of juggling and it might not be right for you if you share a one bedroom apartment on the 12th floor.

And so, We Begin…

AS I DESCRIBED EARLIER, the best way you can start is with a rudimentary practice rig. As long as it's solid and in a safe place where breaking a plate is either very difficult or no real problem, then you are ready to begin.

Spinning the plate

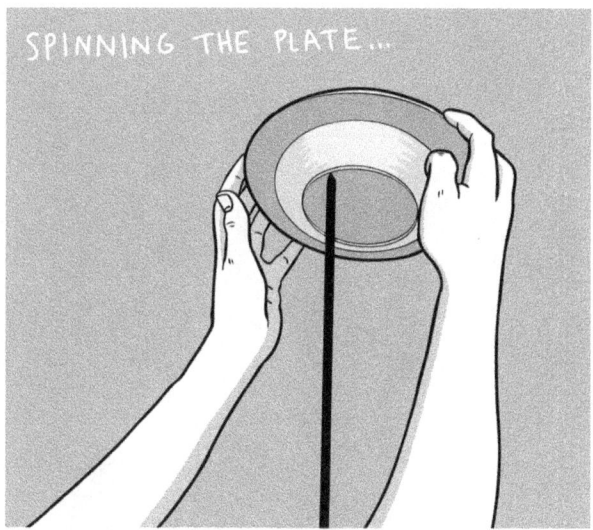

Hold the plate between the fingers of both hands and place it on the tip of the pole (see diagram). Ideally, you should have the point of the stick resting in the ridge of the foot but if it is slightly off, this doesn't matter. It will find the ridge quickly.

Simply enough, one hand goes forward and the other pulls back to spin the plate. Don't do this too hard as the plate is much more likely to fly off. Do it firmly, but under control.

36 | Pottery in Motion:

It doesn't matter which way you spin the plate. I go forward with my right hand and pull back with the left but it's up to you.

Try to push forward and back with equal strength. If you don't, the pole will sway as the plate spins. This will slow the plate down more quickly and, on a full plate rack, it might collide with a neighbouring plate (especially if that one is swaying too).

If a pole does sway, don't panic. Swaying can be corrected as you accelerate the plate so you don't need to stop and start again.

Although it is impractical, a swaying pole with a plate spinning on the end looks very dramatic and unstable. In the long term, you might want to experiment with how much sway you can get away with. It is supposed to look like the edge of a disaster after all.

Accelerating the plate

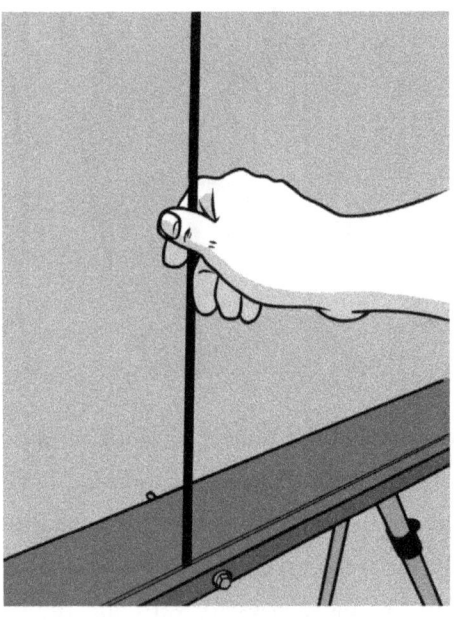

As the plate slows down it will start to wobble and you need to accelerate it back up to full speed by moving the pole. I also refer to this as "rescuing" the plate. Apart from building a workable rack, this is probably the most difficult part of plate spinning.

First of all; DON'T GRAB THE POLE!

If you grip it straight away the plate will most likely fall or become very unstable. Before you accelerate the plate, your hand has to be moving in sympathy with the wobble of the pole. To do this, place your thumb and forefinger round the pole in a very loose pen grip about one third of the way up the stick. Slowly tighten your grip and, as you do so, try to feel the movement of the pole and begin moving your hand at the same speed.

If you do this properly (don't expect to get it straight away) then the pole will be moving your hand, NOT the other way round. Once you reach this state of equilibrium, you can start moving your hand faster to accelerate the plate. Although the tip of the stick will be moving in a circle, the movement with your hands might feel more like a back-and-forth action. The most important thing is the rhythm. If it's slightly off, the tip of the pole will 'skid' on the base of the plate and slow it down or make it unstable.

When you get the hang of this, it will feel very fast and the stick will be a blur of movement.

This sounds like a long and complicated process, but as you get better you will be able to do it very quickly, almost instantaneously. It's like learning to juggle 3 balls or any other skill. It seems complex at first but, with practice, becomes very simple.

Other Techniques

One handed spin

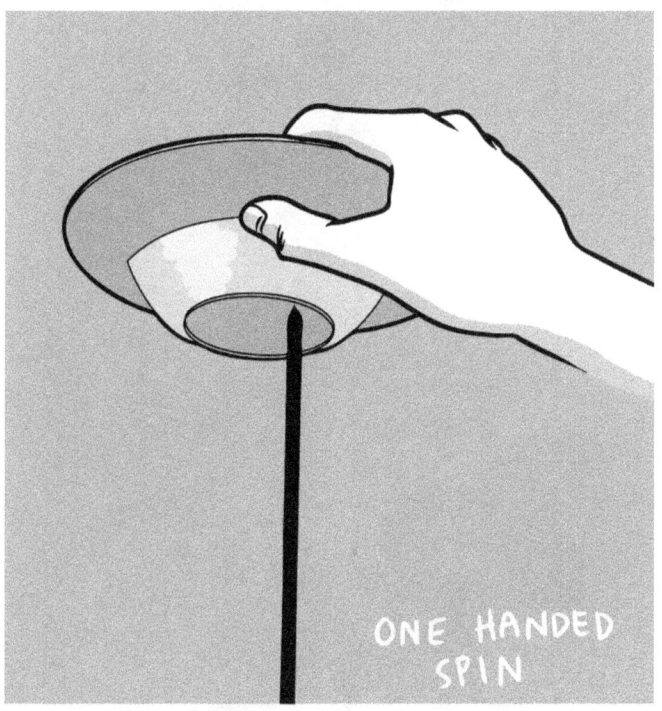

THIS IS ANOTHER TECHNIQUE for getting the plate started (launching the plate). Instead of holding between the fingers of both hands, grip the plate with one hand and place it on the stick with the tip inside the foot ridge closest to your fingers.

Spin the plate with a flick of the wrist in the same direction as you would with two hands. Again, try not to pull back or push forward too much to avoid swaying.

This technique enables you to carry something in your other hand. A stack of plates for example?

Two Handed Acceleration

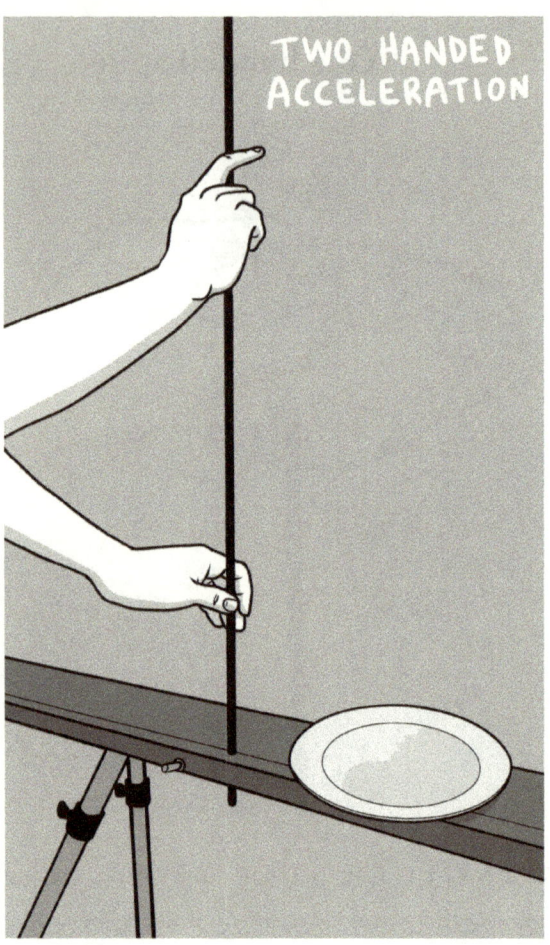

Essentially the same as the technique described above but the accelerating hand goes slightly higher up and the other hand grabs the stick at or near the base. There are a couple of reasons for doing this. If you are using longer, more flexible poles, it helps to stabilise the pole during acceleration and enables you to get to full speed more safely and quickly.

Secondly, from an aesthetic point of view, it makes the performer look a bit more involved with what they are doing which might be preferable when crafting a show. This is very much a matter of opinion.

Taking the Plates Down Again

The safest way to do this is with two hands approaching from below. Place one hand either side of the stick just outside the wobble radius and quickly move your hands upwards scooping the plate off the top of the stick. You can also grab it one handed in much the same way that you would do the one handed spin (above.)

A more dramatic way to do this is to (subtly) slap the pole about a halfway up which will cause the plate to fall straight down. With practice it will fall quite predictably and make you look very cool when you catch it (not guaranteed.)

Troubleshooting

The main parameters affecting plate spinning stability and spin time are...

Pole length
Pole flexibility
Pole tip friction
Pole base stability (rack stability)
Plate diameter
Foot diameter
Foot ridge shape (angle/depth etc)
Plate weight
Plate width
Plate height
Technique

Fine tuning all of these can be a daunting task but hopefully the following will help.

Problems and Possible Solutions

Problem: Plate spins well but falls when accelerated.

Solution 1: The ridge on the plate's foot is not steep or deep enough. Try a different plate/bowl
Solution 2: Base of the plate is wet or covered in condensation
Solution 3: The rescuing/acceleration technique is too rough. Speed up more slowly and smoothly. Try relaxing your arm or changing the way you hold the stick.

Problem: Plate falls when rescued

Solution: This could be the same acceleration problems as above but it could also be the timing of the rescue attempt. At full speed, my plates will spin for over a minute before they fall. This is usually enough but after about 50-55 seconds, the plates reach a point of no return where they spin so slowly and at such an alarming angle, that speeding them up again is a lengthy and highly unreliable process. Ideally, you shouldn't let them get to this stage as accelerating them before this will be much easier. Basically, rescue them sooner.

From a performance point of view however, the more wobble, the better. As your technique improves, this point of no return will be pushed further back until you can easily make some very dramatic saves. I like to practise this by spinning just one plate and letting is slow right down before re-acceleration.

Problem: Plate slows down too quickly.

This could be a technique issue. When you can accelerate a plate properly, your hand should feel relaxed and and you will be shaking it back and forth almost as fast as you can move. This might take a while to learn, so keep practising.

Solution 1: Try to relax your shoulder.

Solution 2: Change the height at which you hold the pole. Only a slight adjustment might do the trick.

Solution 3: Change the angle of your hand and/or wrist. Experiment with holding the stick in different ways.

If that doesn't help, it's also possible that your setup could do with some adjustment.

If you are still at the practice rig stage of development (see the earlier chapter on rig design) it should be easy to make the following changes.

Solution 4: Change the length of the pole. Longer or shorter. Even a difference of a couple of inches can change the spin time.

Solution 5: Make sure the pole is firmly fixed into the base. If there is any play at all between the pole and the table top, the plate will slow more quickly.

Solution 6: Make sure that the rack is steady on the floor and doesn't wobble at all. Adjust the legs or place it on more even ground if need be. Consider weighting it down (again, refer back to the chapter on rig design.)

The problem could also be in your choice of plate. If it's too light, it will slow down more quickly. If the foot is too large or the bowl is too tall, this could also affect the spin time. Most factory made plates will be evenly weighted, but if you are using a more unusual contemporary design, the centre of gravity may not be in the centre of the foot. This won't help either. It might also be time to try adapting the tips of the poles (refer to the notes on "Adapting the Tips" in an earlier chapter.)

Problem: It takes too long to get the plate back up to full speed.

Again, this could be technique and it will improve with practice. Remember, aim to accelerate smoothly and the speed will come in time.
If not…
Solution: Try using plates with a smaller foot diameter.

Big Finish

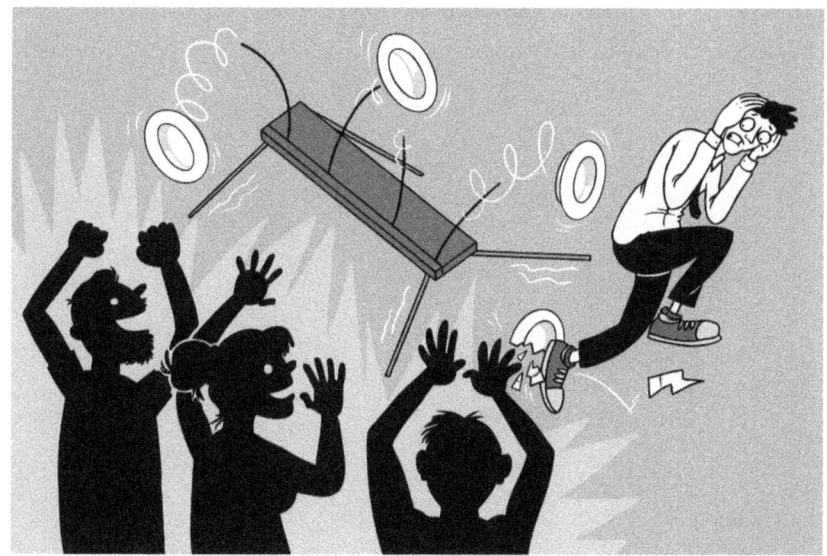

ONE OF MY FIRST plate spinning shows was at a children's festival in a small town in England. I arrived at the venue, carefully set up my plate racks and went out to perform the first of 3 shows that afternoon.

Show number 1 was nerve-racking but it went well and I went into show 2 with renewed confidence. As with the first show, I got all 8 plates spinning and took a bow. Then, at the last minute (to build tension), I ran back to the racks to gather the plates. The first 4 plates were taken down and placed quickly but neatly on the table top. Focusing on the remaining plates, I ran to the second rack and accidentally kicked one of the legs as I arrived sending all four of them crashing to the floor in perfect time with the end of the music.

The crowd went wild and I took another bow. After the show, several people asked if I did that every time. "Of course I do" I told them.

I only had seven plates left for the final show, so I removed one of the sticks and used the empty section of the table top to store all the plates. The final show went well and I learnt two things that day. Unsuccessful plate spinning can be just as entertaining if not more entertaining than a perfect show and… carry more spare plates than you think you need.

Notes on Performance

OK. LET'S JUMP AHEAD a little and assume that you've built yourself a portable rack, found some suitable plates and learnt how to spin them proficiently. Maybe that's enough for you? It is surprisingly good exercise after all. Some of you though, will want to demonstrate your new found skill to the world and perform it somewhere. Exactly how you do that is up to you, but I hope you will find the following advice useful.

We will start with the practical stuff…

Wind

If you are working outdoors, wind will make the plates slow down more quickly. More wind = more slow-down. You may have to adapt your routine to include fewer plates on a windy day.

Transport

Currently, I'm carrying my plate racks in a snowboard bag. This is fine for getting to and from the car but would be difficult on public transport. If you are travelling by plane, a hard case would be better. Hardshell snowboard cases and other long cases are available, but if your plate spinning show is getting you booked abroad, maybe it's time to get something custom made? The case can even be the table top for your plate rack. Dream big, pack small!

I carry my plates in a padded bag designed for a drum of a similar diameter. A piece of corrugated cardboard or foam is placed between each plate. Once again, pack plenty of spares!

Water and Moisture

Don't let the base of the plate get wet. This can happen if the plate gets very cold and is bought into a warmer environment and picks up condensation. If it gets wet and slippery, the stick will skid on the base of the plate making acceleration more difficult and the plate might fall when accelerated too quickly.

Tech Rehearsal

If at all possible, arrive early and set up your plate racks on stage. Make sure they are stable on the floor and mark the position of the legs with tape so that they can be placed quickly and accurately when needed. Store them out of the way backstage.

If you have to set them up away from the stage, plan your route to carry them onstage. My racks are just low enough to get through a doorway. Yours might not be!

Risk Assessment

A lot of venues require a risk assessment. This is especially true for unusual acts that they don't see regularly. I've included my risk assessment for plate spinning at the end of the book. You may wish to add to it or edit it for your own show.

Creating a Show

The classic narrative of a plate spinning routine involves a lot of running around whilst gradually building up the number of plates being spun. When a critical number of plates is reached, another juggling/balancing/manipulation trick is performed in the short window before the spinning plates slow down and fall. The plates are then taken down and the audience (with any luck) goes wild.

This is a formula that works but there is no reason why you have to stick to it. Likewise, there are no guidelines as to how many plates you should spin or how long the show should be. I like to talk during my plate act, most people do the whole thing to music and don't say a word. It's very much up to you.

Remember…

- You are effectively performing one trick with a long build-up. It's almost like setting up a combination juggling trick where you (for example) balance something on your head, spin something on your finger and, finally, juggle with your other hand. It's all a prelude to that final picture.
- It's fun to perform in a top hat and use an old timey Music Hall/Vaudeville theme, but don't feel you have to do it like this.
- Solo juggling/balancing isn't always the best way to fill a large stage but with plate spinning, you can cover a lot more ground. If you use multiple racks, experiment with placing them further apart. This not only fills more space but involves more running around.
- Be wary of looking too relaxed. As you get more comfortable with the props, you might start to appear in control and lose the jeopardy of plate spinning. (On the other hand, you might want to look completely in control and make that style your very own. Again, it's up to you).
- Don't worry about breaking plates. They are a tax write-off!

Tool Kit for Plate Spinning

Consider carrying the following with you when you are travelling with your plate rack.

- Spares (spare plates, a spare pole. If your rack has bolts, screws or other fittings, carry spares of these too.)
- Tools for assembling rack (box spanner, Allen key etc. Depends on your design.)
- Cloth (for drying plates that become damp.)
- Dust pan and brush (be realistic - nobody's perfect!)
- Gaffer tape/Duct tape (generally a good idea for any performer.)
- Level or Spirit Level.

54 | Pottery in Motion:

Risk Assessment - Plate Spinning

Potential hazards -

- Sharp edges of broken china plates
- Falling plates
- Trip hazard caused by legs of plate racks on stage
- Trip hazard caused by legs of plate racks when stored backstage or in the wings

People at risk -

- The performer
- The audience
- Theatre staff

Managing the risks -

- Only doing the routine on a clearly marked stage area, not an open space with passers by
- Not putting the plate racks too close to the edge of the stage
- Making sure the stage management team are ready with a broom after the set
- Making sure there is time to clear the stage before the next act is on (if any)
- Inform children in the audience (if any) not to pick up broken pieces of plate

- Finding a good place to store the racks backstage so they are well out of the way until needed
- Plates might be stored on or under the plate rack so inform everyone backstage of this so they can be careful and avoid if possible

Conclusion

I hope that you find the time and space to explore the possibilities in this book. If not, I hope it at least makes an interesting addition to your bookshelf. Visitors to your home can pick it up and assume you are an eccentric polymath who once ran away with the circus, then they can put it back on the shelf in between David Hasslehoff's autobiography and your 1936 edition of Mrs Beeton's Household Management.

Compared to other forms of juggling and manipulation, plate spinning can be a very big undertaking. You probably have many other things going on in your life and have to attend to those too, giving each one a little attention and then, in turn, moving on to the next until you are maintaining a lot of things at once like you were... erm... I don't know! Busy or something.

Plate spinning has as much scope for re-invention and re-interpretation as any other juggling skill or performing art. It may continue to be celebrated as a traditional act or it may evolve into something entirely new. Exactly how it evolves is up to you.

I considered signing off with something cheesy like "Have a smashing time!" Unfortunately, that is more or less inevitable regardless of what I say. Instead, I shall simply wish you the very best of luck.

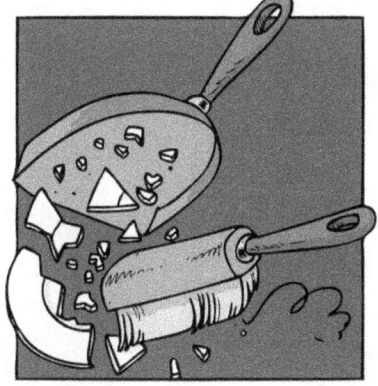

58 | Pottery in Motion:

SPECIAL THANKS

The following people, listed in alphabetical order, offered help in researching, editing, and testing this book.

Liam Bradley
David Cain
Andy Gray
Rob Horsman
Sophie Lewis
Ian Marchant
Simon Merton
Winston Plowes
Sorrel Sparks
Jon Udry
Phillippe Viel
Thom Wall
Maya Zuckerman

About the Author

Plate spinner, juggler, comedian, children's entertainer, teacher, yo-yo salesman and hand model Sam Veale, has been a full time performer for over 20 years. He began juggling in the early 1990s but didn't learn plate spinning until much more recently. At the time there was little or no published information about plate spinning. This book hopes to plug that gap.

He lives in Surrey in England with his wife and two daughters.

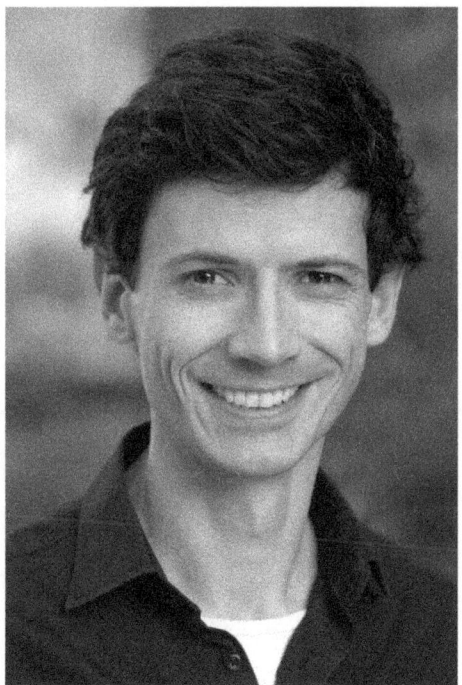

Photograph by Matt Hennem

Other Books by Modern Vaudeville Press

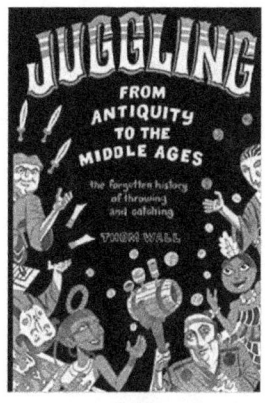

Juggling: From Antiquity to the Middle Ages
Thom Wall
ISBN 978-0-578-41084-5

As with dance, so with juggling—the moment that the performer finishes the routine, their act ceases to exist beyond the memory of the audience. There is no permanent record of what transpired, so studying the ancient roots of juggling is fraught with difficulty. Using the records that do exist, juggling appears to have emerged around the world in cultures independent of one another in the ancient past. Paintings in Egypt from 2000 BCE show jugglers engaged in performance. Stories from the island nation of Tonga place juggling's creation with their goddess of the underworld—a figure who has guarded a cave since time immemorial. Juggling games and rituals are pervasive in isolated Inuit cultures in northern Canada and Greenland. Though the earliest representation of juggling is 4,000 years old, the practice is surely much older—in the same way that humans were doubtlessly singing and dancing long before the first bone flute was created.

This book is an attempt to catalogue this tangible history of juggling in human culture. It is the story of juggling, represented in art and writing from around the world, across time. Although much has been written about modern jugglers–specific performers, their props, and their routines–little has been said about those who first developed the

64 | Pottery in Motion:

craft. As juggling enters a golden age in the internet era, Juggling: From Antiquity to the Middle Ages offers a look into the past—to the origins of our art form.

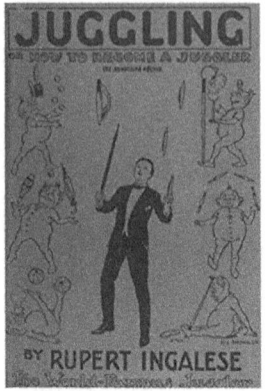

Juggling - or how to become a juggler (the annotated edition)
Rupert Ingalese, Thom Wall
ISBN 978-1-7339712-0-1

Rupert Ingalese, born Paul Wingrave, was a British juggler who worked in the first half of the 1900s, both as a juggler and as a producer and manager of variety shows across England. In 1917, he published the very first "learn to juggle" book, teaching in detail the methods used to learn traditional toss juggling, as well as a variety of more esoteric juggling skills.

This book offers complete annotations that add context to Ingalese's writing, as well as asides that explain the work of other jugglers in the same time period.

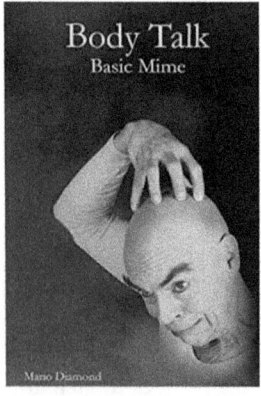

Body Talk: Basic Mime
Mario Diamond
ISBN 978-1-7339712-1-8

Body Talk is Mario Diamond's detailed introduction to the art of mime. Body axes, illusions, and exploratory games are laid out accessibly for any learner.

The Midwest Book Review calls this book "...a highly recommended 'must' for any theater or drama reference collection and for producers and actors who want to translate mime's basics to better acting and cognitive results."

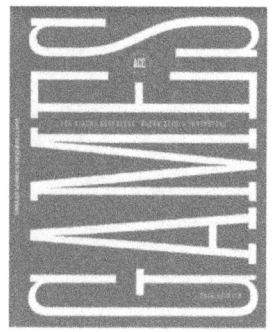

Games for Circus Educators, Organizers & Innovators
American Youth Circus Organization, compiled by Lucy Little
ISBN 978-1-7339712-2-5

With over 100 games organized for optimal use in cooperative movement based settings, this is a must have for every circus school, teaching artist, and arts education program! Games are organized by age, number of participant, energy level, and social/emotional learning outcome, and also includes special notes for working with a variety of populations that may require adaptation or modifications to each game.

www.ingramcontent.com/pod-product-compliance
Lightning Source LLC
Chambersburg PA
CBHW020303030426
42336CB00010B/884